STUFF EVERY

CANNABISSEUR

SHOULD KNOW

Stuff Every
Cannabisseur
Should Know

by Marc Luber

QUIRK BOOKS
PHILADELPHIA

Copyright © 2019 by Quirk Productions, Inc.

All rights reserved. Except as authorized under U.S. copyright law, no part of this book may be reproduced in any form without written permission from the publisher.

Library of Congress Cataloging in Publication Number: 2018964793

ISBN: 978-1-68369-134-1

Printed in China

Typeset in Adobe Garamond, Brandon Grotesque, and Akzidenz-Grotesk BQ

Designed by Aurora Parlagreco
Illustrations by Lucy Engelman
Production management by John J. McGurk

Quirk Books
215 Church Street
Philadelphia, PA 19106
quirkbooks.com

10 9 8 7 6 5 4 3 2 1

To the legalization of marijuana

LIVING YOUR BEST CANNABISSEUR LIFE

THE CULTURE OF CANNABIS

FURTHER READING

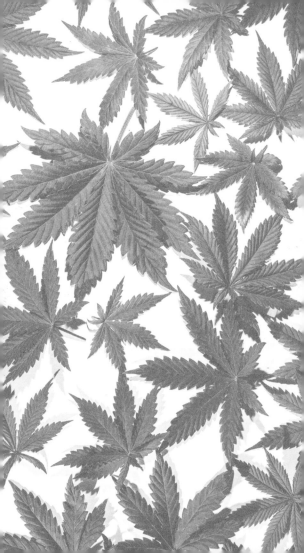

What Is a Cannabisseur?

CAN·NA·BIS·SEUR

n: **1.** cannabis expert, especially one who understands and admires all things related to cannabis and the culture surrounding its popularity and use. **2.** an expert who understands the many benefits of marijuana and can navigate the vast landscape that has been created from one incredible plant.

Marijuana is one of the most wonderful gifts that nature has to offer. Long before it took root in modern popular culture, cannabis had a long history spanning the globe. Evidence of its commercial usage extends back to 10,000 BCE, and since then nearly every major civilization has found some use for this powerful drug, either recreationally, medically, and spiritually/religiously.

The criminalization of cannabis began in the mid-nineteenth century, and for most of the twentieth century, the herb's sale and usage was conducted behind closed doors. Yet it is undeniable that, in recent decades, recreational and medical marijuana use has made a major comeback and is growing in popularity—and legality—around the world.

Now that marijuana use is becoming destigmatized and decriminalized, it's high time that we approach this mood-altering substance with the same level of consideration, education, exploration, and experimentation as we do wine, beer, and liquor. In order to do this, we need to cultivate the cannabis-equivalent of sommeliers: experts who can help casual users and the merely curious navigate the big wide world of weed.

In short: it's time for the rise of the cannabisseur.

A self-proclaimed cannabisseur, I have written this book as a guide to help potheads grow into their own expertise. Think of this as a pocket-sized crash course in cannabis certification. I'll take you through a bit of history as well as the usage, applications, effects, and culture of weed. I'll also offer you some fun how-tos to take your toke to the next level.

Though some people are able to grow, buy, or use marijuana legally, it is important to remember that marijuana possession is illegal in many parts of the United States and in many countries around the world. This book is meant to educate and entertain, but I strongly recommended that you always follow local laws regarding marijuana. The drug affects everyone differently, and a single user can experience varying effects depending on factors such as how long ago you ate a meal, what kind of marijuana you're consuming, and the circumstances in which you're enjoying it. Always exercise good judgment with weed, and be sure to familiarize yourself with its effects (see page 39) as well as the differences between smoking, eating, and using concentrates (pages 53–63). We recommend discussing your usage with your doctor, in case other drugs you take could interact adversely with it. The resources on page 143 also offer a wealth of useful information.

That said, let's spend a little time expanding your mind and exploring all the stuff every cannabisseur should know.

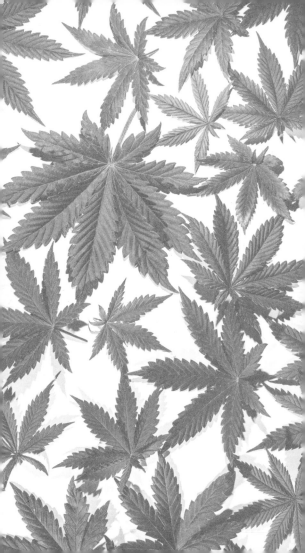

Cannabis
Basics

Terms Every Cannabisseur Should Know

Baked: The feeling one experiences when incredibly high on marijuana.

Binger: Filling a chamber of a water pipe with marijuana smoke and inhaling all of it at once. Also known as a *bong hit*.

Blunt: A hollowed-out cigar filled with marijuana.

Bong: A device used for smoking weed and other substances. Many variations of bongs exist, but the simplest consists of a basin, tube (or chamber), bowl, and stem. The basin portion is filled with water, which filters the smoke and minimizes the ash and tar that reach the user's mouth.

Bowl: A pipe in which marijuana is placed to be smoked.

Bud: The flower of the marijuana plant, which contains cannabinoids such as THC, CBD, CBG, and THCV.

Cannabinoid: A chemical compound either derived from, or synthetically produced to mimic, the naturally occurring compounds in the cannabis plant, which acts on specific receptors in the human body. These include compounds with psychoactive properties, namely THC, as well as those that can influence appetite, memory, and other functions without altering mood.

Cannabis: Genus of a tall flowering plant originating in Central Asia that is cultivated for both drug and nondrug uses. Cannabis is commonly used interchangeably with the term *marijuana*.

Canoeing: When a joint burns more on one side than another, giving it the look of a canoe. This can be a waste of marijuana and is generally caused when marijuana is not ground before being added to a joint, or if it is unevenly spaced in the joint, or by rolling a joint too loosely or too tight.

Chronic: Very high quality weed. This term is generally attributed to the rapper Snoop Dogg and was later used by record producer and rapper Dr. Dre as the title of his debut album. According to Snoop Dogg, he misheard the term "hydroponic," a means by which good marijuana is grown, as "hydrochronic." He later shortened the term to *chronic*. The world is a better place because nobody told Snoop he was saying it wrong.

Concentrates: Cannabis-derived products that contain concentrated amounts of THC, such as kief, shatter, wax, and oils. These tend to be significantly more potent than marijuana flowers and are made by extracting THC from the plant using various methods incorporating heat, pressure, and solvents.

Cone: A joint made in a conical shape, which allows it to be filled with more marijuana and to last longer than a standard joint.

Dabbing: A method of consuming certain concentrates by heating them on a surface at an extremely high temperature before inhaling them. Doing so requires specialized equipment and can be dangerous if not performed properly. The physical effects of dabbing can be significantly more intense than those of other forms of consumption.

Dank: Like chronic, another term used to designate high-quality weed. Although you may smoke dank weed with your friends, overusing this term will leave you smoking it alone in your dank basement.

Dispensary: A retail store where marijuana can be legally purchased, generally only with cash.

Edibles: This umbrella term refers to all THC products that can be eaten. Though the pot brownie may be the most famous edible, today's edibles can be candies, teas or other beverages, and almost anything you can make using ordinary vegetable oil.

Grinder: A tool used to break down marijuana buds into small pieces to make them more manageable for use in joints, bowls, edible oil, etc. Grinders can be purchased at specialty stores or online.

Hashish: A type of cannabis concentrate made by condensing kief; also known as hash.

Head shop: A specialty store that stocks bongs, bowls, grinders, vaporizers, and other drug paraphernalia. Note that such establishments may operate where marijuana is illegal, so always use discretion and never mention weed when shopping.

Hemp: Term referring to nonpsychoactive varieties of *Cannabis sativa*, aka those containing less than 1 percent THC. Hemp comes from the same cannabis species as marijuana but differs in its genetics as well as use, chemical makeup, and growing methods.

Herb: Slang term referring to the dried and cured marijuana flowers that are smoked.

Hybrids: Strains that are bred from the two main species of the cannabis plant, *Cannabis indica* and *Cannabis sativa*, used in various proportions. Blending the two can produce a plant that offers the specific desired effects from each species. For example, a hybrid might provide a person with pain relief while also keeping them alert and awake.

Indica: One of the two major strains of the cannabis plant, it is thought that indica provides a relaxing and mellow high. This strain is often used as a sleep aid, pain reliever, or appetite stimulator. The high from indica tends to affect the entire body, as opposed to just a head high. The cannabisseur knows that indica generally means "in da couch."

Joint: A rolled marijuana cigarette. This is the most traditional means of smoking cannabis. May be referred to as a spliff, fattie, doobie, or simply a "j."

Kief: Tiny sticky crystals that coat the surface of marijuana flowers. Kief can be easily removed from the buds by using a grinder; the ground buds remain in the strainer portion of the grinder while the kief settles in the bottom storage portion, to be used later. These crystals are the plant's defense against herbivores that might eat the flowers; ironically, kief works by producing an intense psychoactive experience for the animal, preventing it from wanting to eat more. (That doesn't seem to work for many of us humans.)

Kush: A popular variety of marijuana generally derived from an indica strain of cannabis.

Marijuana: The dried resinous flower buds and leaves of the female cannabis plant that contain high levels of THC and can be smoked, vaped, or eaten for their intoxicating effect.

Nug: The main pieces, or nuggets, of marijuana buds that have been dried and cured. The cannabisseur refers to nugs as those pieces of higher-quality marijuana that have the right color and crystallized appearance and that don't contain seeds.

Pinner: A very skinny joint, generally made for one or two people to share; may be the result of a shortage of marijuana supply or simply the preference of a conscientious and frugal cannabisseur.

Sativa: One of two major strains of the cannabis plant, sativa has the impact of a more uplifting and euphoric high. This strain is often used for promoting creativity and increasing energy and alertness. The high from the sativa strain is generally a head high rather than a full-body high.

Schwag: Term for poor-quality marijuana. The cannabisseur avoids schwag at all costs.

Shatter: A hard, glasslike extract from the cannabis plant that can contain as much as 90 percent THC.

Shotgun: A small hole on a pipe that's covered while marijuana is burned; when a hit is taken, the shotgun is uncovered to allow fresh air to enter the pipe and clear the chamber of smoke.

Skunk: Descriptor for the scent of quality marijuana. Surprisingly, the smell of very good weed closely resembles that of a skunk's defense spray.

Spliff: A type of joint generally made with a mixture of tobacco and marijuana when you don't have enough weed to fill a joint.

Sticky Icky: Slang term for high-quality marijuana as indicated by its sticky, resinous surface. The resin is produced by trichome glands on the surface of the cannabis flower. Snoop Dogg made the term famous in the song "Still Dre" on Dr. Dre's album *2001*: "Some of that real sticky icky icky . . . Oooh wee! Put it in the air."

Stoned: The intense, euphoric feeling achieved when you use the right amount of marijuana. Perhaps a step below being baked, but it's not a contest, people—just enjoy the ride.

Strains: Varieties of cannabis plants. There are two primary strains of cannabis, sativa and indica, and new and unique hybrid strains are created all the time by breeding these plants together.

THC: Tetrahydrocannabinol, aka the chemical compound found in the cannabis plant that is responsible for its psychoactive effects. When marijuana is used, THC attaches to cannabinoid receptors in the brain largely associated with thinking, memory, pleasure, time perception, and coordination.

Vaporizer: Any electronic device designed to inhale a heated liquid or plant material without burning it; also known as a vape pen or, simply, "vape." Vaporizers were first developed for use with tobacco as a means to enjoy it without the dangerous effects of burning nicotine (found in cigarettes) or inhaling smoke. Today, vaporizers are used to heat various forms of marijuana, including wax and oils.

Wax: A type of concentrate that is extracted from the marijuana buds using propane, butane, or another solvent. Wax typically has a soft and thick consistency reminiscent of a melted candle. Particularly soft wax is referred to as "budder," while harder varieties are known as "crumble."

Weed: Synonym for marijuana.

A Brief History of Cannabis

The many uses of cannabis have been known and appreciated for centuries. Let's take a look at the rich history of this versatile plant.

Ca. 10,000 BCE: First evidence of cannabis usage. Central Asian cultures cultivate the indigenous hemp plant to make pottery, rope, and fabric.

Ca. 8,000 BCE: Cannabis becomes an important raw material for essential trade goods like clothing, shoes, rope, and paper in China, Japan, and Korea.

3,000–2,000 BCE: The Chinese emperor Shennong refers to cannabis for the first time in recorded history in 2727 BCE. Cannabis is steeped as a tea to help treat an array of illnesses, including malaria and gout. A thousand years later, it is used for medicinal and religious purposes in India as well. Records and documents indicate prevalent cannabis use by Chinese physicians by the turn of the first century CE.

1100s: Hashish (aka hash) is introduced to the Muslim world as an edible, beginning in Bahrain and Iraq and spreading to the Egyptian Sufis. Through exploration and trade, cannabis cultivation spreads to Africa, via Arab and Hindu travelers, and the Western world.

1545: Spain cultivates industrial hemp in Chile, marking the plant's introduction to the New World.

Early 1600s: Hemp plants grow wildly and successfully in the American South and are used to create rope, paper, and cloth products. Virginia considers hemp a form of currency and passes a law in 1619 that requires all farms in the colony to grow it. Once King Cotton takes over the South, the need for hemp diminishes greatly.

Mid-1800s: As hemp production dwindles in the U.S., medical cannabis becomes more popular. In the Portuguese colony of Brazil, enslaved people use cannabis for its psychoactive properties, which triggers the first known restriction of cannabis usage. Meanwhile, in British colonies like Jamaica, indentured servants from India introduce seedlings of *Cannabis indica*. (Ganja, which is a widely used term for marijuana in Jamaica, comes from the Hindu and Sanskrit words meaning "hemp.") The British Commonwealth becomes concerned about the use of ganja by laborers in various colonies and takes steps to outlaw it.

1913: Jamaica outlaws marijuana with the passage of the Ganja Law. The British Commonwealth and many of its colonies follow suit.

1914: Recreational marijuana use, which was likely brought to the United States by refugees fleeing the Mexican Revolution, is banned in El Paso, Texas, as a legal attack on immigration. El Paso is the first city to pass an ordinance against marijuana use.

1937: After various states outlaw the consumption of marijuana, beginning with California, the Marijuana Tax Act criminalizes the sale of the plant, effectively banning it from U.S. soil.

1970: The Marijuana Tax Act is replaced by the Controlled Substances Act and signed into law by President Richard Nixon. It establishes a federal drug policy that ranks substances according to their potential for addiction and degree of danger. President Nixon's Schafer Commission declares that marijuana should *not* be classified as a Schedule I drug, the most restrictive category, and even doubts its designation as an illicit substance. Disregarding this recommendation, President Nixon allows cannabis to be placed in Schedule I, along with drugs like LSD, mescaline, and heroin. As of 2019, it remains a Schedule I controlled substance according to U.S. federal law.

1972: The Netherlands updates the classification of marijuana to be considered less dangerous than before and lightens the penalties imposed on possession of the drug. Within four years, some coffee shops had begun providing local residents the option to purchase and use cannabis products on store property.

> Although many people today consider Amsterdam to be one of the most weed-positive cities in the world, recreational marijuana use is illegal in the Netherlands. (Medical use is not.) In some parts of the country, coffee shop purchases are limited to residents of the Netherlands; the city of Amsterdam has a more lenient policy that allows tourists to purchase and smoke marijuana on store property as well.

1996: California, which was the first U.S. state to outlaw cannabis, becomes the first state to legalize medical marijuana. Other states, including Nevada, Vermont, and Washington, follow California's lead.

2015: Marijuana is decriminalized in Jamaica. Jamaicans may cultivate, possess, and use the drug in small amounts. Jamaica continues to evolve its laws to become a more pot-friendly destination, and policies are constantly changing.

2019: As of the publication of this book, marijuana has been legalized in ten U.S. states and Washington, D.C., and many states have either legalized medical marijuana, decriminalized recreational marijuana, or both. It remains illegal in thirteen states. Globally, Canada and Georgia have legalized weed for recreational and medical use. Argentina, Australia, Chile, Colombia, Croatia, the Czech Republic, Denmark, Greece, Israel, Italy, Luxembourg, Macedonia, Malta, the Netherlands, Norway, Peru, Poland, Portugal, Sri Lanka, Switzerland, Uruguay, Vanuatu, and Zimbabwe have legalized medical marijuana, and other countries have decriminalized recreational marijuana.

How Cannabis Is Grown

Cannabis was cultivated naturally outdoors for centuries, but in recent years a number of factors have led to a huge wave of indoor cultivation. Considering the climate requirements for growing cannabis, the most successful outdoor growth will take place within 35 degrees of the equator. The amount of daylight the plants get is also a critical factor that further limits the potential locales that successfully produce plants with a high quantity of THC.

Perhaps the most limiting factor for where marijuana can be grown outdoors is that its cultivation is illegal in many parts of the world.

The global high demand for potent quality products and increasing decriminalization have opened new opportunities for indoor cannabis farmers. Indoor facilities allow growers to experiment with cross-breeding and to meticulously control the variables of temperature, light, humidity, growth medium (typically soil), and water, allowing farmers to produce higher quality plants more quickly than is possible with natural growth. They can also offer highly specific strains to demanding consumers.

Cannabis growth can be broken down into four stages that are similar to the growth of other flowering plants.

Stage 1: Germination

In the first week after planting, the cannabis seed will begin to sprout, and a small root will sprout, growing downward. Soon after, the embryonic seed leaves, known as cotyledons, will begin to emerge aboveground in search of light. Like its eventual end user, the plant yearns to get higher (For more on seeds, see page 30.)

Stage 2: Seedling

In the subsequent 2 to 4 weeks, the plant is most vulnerable to significant changes in light, moisture, or humidity. Toward the end of this phase, the leaves will begin to form that familiar fanlike shape we all know and love.

Stage 3: Vegetative

No, this is not the phase you enter after doing your first gravity bong hit. This is the 1 to 2 months when the plant grows the most and generally requires the most light. The plant will have seven sets of leaves and the sex will be revealed during this phase. Female plants, which are more desirable, tend to be shorter and will produce buds without seeds.

Stage 4: Flowering

The final phase of the growth process, which generally lasts 6 to 12 weeks, is when the flowering buds are fully formed. The plant tends to require less light during this time, and the overall size of the plant increases significantly. Now is when trichomes appear on the surface of the buds in order to protect the plant from animals or insects looking for a bite to eat. The resin they produce contains the highest concentration of THC and cannabinol and gives the buds their crystalized exterior.

The Harvest

After the final stage of growing, when the trichomes appear cloudy and reddish, it's time to gather the crop. During harvest, the buds are removed from the plant and are dried in an environment of lower humidity and darkness. The dry buds must then be cured in an airtight container for about 4 more weeks before they are ready to be consumed. If cured properly, the buds can gain potency.

It's a long journey from seed to weed, but any cannabisseur will tell you it is well worth the wait.

A NOTE ABOUT SEEDS

The best cannabis is all about genetics. Over time, growers have selected the best seedlings from each crop and used them to create ideal strains. The characteristics that growers look for when determining which seeds are better than others include gender (only female plants can produce cannabis buds), color, yield, growing time, flavor, and, of course, consumer appeal.

Growers can produce plants from the preferred feminized seeds and cultivate them to produce specific strains again and again. Once the seedlings have been selected, it's time to start growing.

Know Your Strains

The two species of the cannabis plant produced for consumption are *Cannabis sativa* and *Cannabis indica*. The high induced from sativa strains is uplifting, energizing, and even euphoric; this is the strain you'd use to enhance your ability to focus on a creative project. The indica strain induces a high that's more mellow and relaxing. As opposed to the "head high" caused by sativa, indica typically affects the entire body, making it useful as a sleep aid and pain reliever. Indica plants tend to be shorter, with wide leaves and dense buds. Sativa plants are typically taller, with thin leaves and feathery buds. (Illustrations on page 32.)

Stemming from these is a large variety of strains developed and named by growers based on the appearance, smell, or taste of the buds. Strains number in the hundreds, and growers continue to experiment with producing new variations. Strains are usually categorized as sativa, indica, or hybrid, depending on the plant's origins. The effects can vary widely, so knowing what effect you desire is your principal concern when choosing a strain.

Perhaps the most popular cannabis strain, Haze, was created by the pair of eponymous brothers in the 1970s, when they crossed two high-quality sativa strains from Colombia and Mexico. The Haze brothers took the very best females from this hybrid and crossed them a second time with a southern Indian landrace strain (locally adapted variety). Again, they took the best females from this hybrid and crossed them with a landrace strain from Thailand. The results of their efforts can be found in marijuana plants around the world.

A sampling of popular strains, with their main identifying characteristics, appears on pages 33–35.

SATIVA   INDICA

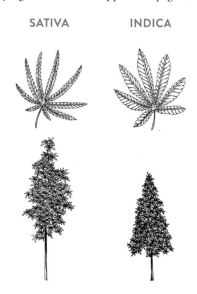

POPULAR SATIVA STRAINS

STRAIN	CHARACTERISTICS
Acapulco Gold	High THC content, orange hairs, difficult to find
Lamb's Bread	Sticky green buds, high-energy effect
Maui Wowie	Sweet tropical flavor, uplifting high
Purple Haze	Lavender-hued buds, social/uplifting high
Sour Diesel	Pungent odor, energetic cerebral high
Super Lemon Haze	Citrus odor, giggly euphoric high

POPULAR INDICA STRAINS

STRAIN	CHARACTERISTICS
Afghan Kush	Very relaxing high, easy to find, beware of munchies
Blueberry	Colorful buds, high THC content, long-lasting calming high
Bubba Kush	Sedative high, rich coffee flavor
Grape Ape	Carefree stress-relieving high, grape aroma
Northern Lights	Pungent spicy aroma, pure indica, full-body high

POPULAR HYBRID STRAINS

STRAIN	CHARACTERISTICS
Blue Dream	Sativa dominant, sweet berry aroma, high THC content
Girl Scout Cookies	Known as GSC, orange hairs, euphoric and relaxing high
Juicy Fruit	Multicolored buds, citrus aroma, predominantly cerebral high
OG Kush	Parent to a large number of strains, euphoric high, difficult to find
Pineapple Express	Fresh tropical aroma, energetic high

THC versus CBD

Both tetrahydrocannabinol (THC) and cannabidiol (CBD) are natural compounds in the cannabis plant. THC is primarily extracted from the buds or flowers, where it is most concentrated, but it can also be found in trace amounts throughout the plant. CBD is primarily extracted from the portions of the plant that contain only those trace amounts of THC.

Both of these compounds affect the endocannabinoid system in the human body, which is the network that facilitates communication between the brain and other parts of the body in order to regulate functions including appetite, memory, stress, pain response, sleep, and even female reproduction. Such communication occurs between neurotransmitters and cannabinoid receptors found throughout the central and peripheral nervous systems. When THC or CBD enters the bloodstream (either through the lungs or stomach, depending on how it is consumed), the compound binds to cannabinoid receptors and activates them.

Both compounds have been shown to exert positive health benefits on the body through these receptors, but only THC provides the psychoactive effects sought by recreational marijuana users. It is for this reason that THC is present in all varieties of marijuana herb, edibles, and concentrates that are consumed to elicit the high or euphoric feeling commonly associated with marijuana. Although both substances have medicinal uses, the psychoactive properties of THC explain why it is more tightly restricted in many parts of the world than CBD, which is legal to have and use almost anywhere.

The high that comes from absorbing THC into the bloodstream has been known for centuries, if not millennia; the use of CBD in oils and other products is a more recent phenomenon. CBD was first isolated from the cannabis plant in 1940, and only recently have its medicinal purposes for humans and pets entered the mainstream consciousness.

CBD is commonly sold as an oil-based product that may be smoked or absorbed through the mouth or skin. It can also be found, in various edible forms, as an alternative to THC in medical dispensaries. Aside from drowsiness and a potential drop in blood pressure, there are no known significant side effects to CBD use.

CBD is commonly used to treat anxiety and pain associated with multiple sclerosis and epilepsy in children, as well as to stimulate appetite. Research continues to seek out other health benefits. CBD's nonpsychoactive properties make it a viable option for people seeking remedies for health issues but don't want, or can't tolerate, the high associated with regular marijuana use. The U.S. Food and Drug Administration has approved a CBD-based product: Epidiolex, an oral solution used to treat seizures and a rare serious form of epilepsy called Dravet syndrome.

The Effects of Using Cannabis

The cannabisseur should be aware of the positive and negative consequences of getting high—and how to deal with each effect.

MUNCHIES

People who use marijuana recreationally are no doubt familiar with the sudden onset of hunger experienced after getting high. THC interacts with the hypothalamus, which is the area of the brain that controls appetite. THC also affects receptors in the olfactory system, making the smell and taste of food more intense, which means that bag of Cheetos is now more irresistibly delicious than ever before. Weed smokers are likely to experience unique cravings for food, from sweet to salty and everything in between. For medical marijuana users, an increase in appetite can be a nice effect, but the discerning cannabisseur might want to keep healthy snacks on hand to avoid unwanted extra pounds.

LAUGHTER

A favorite effect of smoking cannabis is the tendency to make the user laugh, often at ridiculous things that might not be funny to a person who isn't high. Attending a comedy show, watching funny movies, or just hanging out with good friends can be so much fun when we're high. Although the science is largely unproven, the likely culprit here is THC's influence on the left temporal and right frontal lobes of the brain—areas that are associated with laughter. This effect of marijuana explains its medicinal use for the treatment of anxiety and depression. Whatever the reason, the cannabisseur knows that laughter is good for the soul. Embrace it and enjoy the fun!

MEMORY AND TIME PERCEPTION

Remember the character Jeff Spicoli from the 1982 film *Fast Times at Ridgemont High*? How about classic scenes of forgetfulness from movies like *Ted*, *Super Troopers*, and *Dazed and Confused*? Although recreational cannabis use will not turn you into a hippie surfer, it will likely affect your short-term memory and perception of time while you are under its influence. It is not uncommon to forget what you were just talking about, drift off in thought during a conversation, or feel like you have been doing something for an hour that has in fact taken less than ten minutes. Generally these effects are harmless and add a bit of humorous uncertainty to your overall experience. The cannabisseur knows not to overdo it and understands that scientists are continuing to study the long-term implications of THC on memory.

PARANOIA

Most weed smokers have had at least one experience with feeling paranoid when getting high. Such experiences can vary greatly depending on the amount of cannabis in one's system, the manner in which it was consumed, and the environment. Some users argue that edibles elicit a stronger feeling of paranoia, whereas others experience nothing of the sort. For most people, paranoia is a rare side effect that passes quickly with the right distraction. Until you know your own tolerance of and tendency for this side effect, start with small amounts of marijuana and gradually build up to a level that provides your desired effect. The cannabisseur always remembers to take slow, deep breaths in through the nose and exhale out through the mouth to help relax when feeling paranoid during a high. Try to relax your mind and body, and this too shall pass.

BLOODSHOT EYES

Red and squinty eyes are a clear indication that someone is stoned. The cause of bloodshot eyes is likely THC's ability to lower blood pressure, which affects veins and capillaries in the eyes. In fact, for this reason marijuana is prescribed for patients with glaucoma, because it has been shown to help relieve ocular pressure. As for why it's hard to keep our eyes open when we're high, the science is a little less clear. Some leading theories suggest that it is caused by the body's reaction to dry eyes, sensitivity to light, or relaxed eyelid muscles during a high. The cannabisseur always remembers to have eye drops handy in case of bloodshot eyes resulting from marijuana use.

Using Cannabis Recreationally

Marijuana is most commonly used for recreational purposes. Some choose it as an alternative to alcohol as a means to relax or enjoy time with friends. Others are drawn to it as a way of self-medicating for physical or emotional concerns. And its popularity is on the rise.

So why do so many people choose to smoke weed rather than using other controlled substances? Most people whose drug of choice is marijuana believe it should not be a controlled substance at all. Unlike heroin and other Schedule I drugs, marijuana has a virtually nonexistent chance of overdose, numerous pleasurable physical effects, and no proven addictive properties.

Compared to alcohol, the most common recreationally used substance, marijuana has numerous advantages. Ever tried to have a conversation with someone after a bout of heavy drinking? How about just trying to function normally without slurring your words or being able to walk a straight line? And then there's the next morning's hangover that leaves you desperately searching for water, headache remedies, and food to absorb what is exuding from your pores. Other serious risks include alcohol poisoning and even death. By contrast, many folks who smoke weed find that they are able to function normally, participate in conversations, and walk a perfectly straight line, if that's what you're into. Even better, there is virtually no possibility of a hangover associated with marijuana use. While users could potentially become sick from overdoing it, such adverse effects hardly compare to the downsides of drinking alcohol excessively.

Medical Uses of Cannabis

Many health organizations, including the American Medical Association and the American Academy of Family Physicians, agree that marijuana has some legitimate medical uses. Experts have identified two active chemicals from the plant that have real-world applications. CBD seems to affect the brain without producing a high, and THC possesses pain-relieving qualities. (See page 36 for more about CBD and THC and the differences between these compounds.)

Marijuana has been shown in research studies to help with the following medical conditions.

Chronic pain: Pain management is the most commonly requested and prescribed usage for medical marijuana. Specific applications include arthritis, Parkinson's disease, multiple sclerosis, and pain associated with various autoimmune disorders.

Insomnia: Indica strains of marijuana have been shown to reduce the duration of REM sleep, which results in fewer dreams. This can also mean fewer nightmares, which makes it useful in the treatment of posttraumatic stress disorder (PTSD).

Glaucoma: Marijuana seems to decrease the pressure inside the eye for short periods of time.

Anxiety: There appears to be a "sweet spot" in which a person can smoke to relax, although anxiety can increase with further use. Specific treatments include PTSD and generalized anxiety disorder.

Chemotherapy: Marijuana has been shown to mitigate the side effects of chemotherapy, increasing appetite and reducing pain and nausea.

Cancer: Studies performed on mice and in cell cultures have shown that CBD can prevent the spread of cancer. There's hope that with more testing, these effects can be replicated in humans.

In a time when conventional medical treatments often consist of various prescription medications, many people have turned to alternative health options. Dependency and addiction to Ambien, Zoloft, and any number of opioid medications have left us seeking natural remedies such as cannabis.

The benefits, risks, and side effects are constantly being researched. Refrain from self-medicating, and consult your physician before making any decisions about medical marijuana use. Though health professionals have mixed views on medical marijuana, many doctors are embracing it, staying on top of trends, and constantly revisiting their stance on prescribing it to their patients.

If you are embarrassed to speak to your physician about medical marijuana for fear of being judged or criticized, try approaching the subject generally, by asking about their professional opinion and thoughts on the subject. You can also state that you consider your medical practitioner a partner in your health care, that you consider medical marijuana a potential treatment option, and that you expect your doctor to be educated and informed about its uses.

Sparking Creativity with Cannabis

Despite the stigma still attached to marijuana use, a wide range of entrepreneurs, artists, designers, and innovators have acknowledged it as a means to boost creativity. Researchers continue to investigate whether marijuana in fact increases creativity or, rather, if creative people are more open to the idea of smoking marijuana than are other individuals.

Studies have found that the increase in dopamine in the brain resulting from marijuana use can lower inhibitions and reduce anxiety. This relaxed state may allow users to see things differently and encourage new behaviors across a variety of academic and creative disciplines, as illustrated by the following iconic creators.

Politics: U.S. founding father James Monroe and John F. Kennedy, the country's thirty-fifth president, are rumored to have used the drug. (Helping establish a democratic nation ranks pretty high on the creativity scale, if you ask us.)

Science and medicine: Pulitzer Prize winning American astronomer Carl Sagan smoked marijuana and was an advocate for its legalization for medical purposes. William Brooke O'Shaughnessy, a nineteenth-century

Irish doctor and scientist, treated patients with cannabis and is considered to have been integral in introducing the drug to Western medicine.

Literature: Renowned British playwright William Shakespeare may have used cannabis. In 2015 traces of the drug were detected on tobacco pipe fragments found on his property in Stratford-on-Avon. Was it weed, or not the weed: that is the question.

Industry and business: Famous innovators like Apple cofounder Steve Jobs, longtime Microsoft CEO Bill Gates, and Ben Cohen and Jerry Greenfield (of Ben and Jerry's ice cream) are all known to have used marijuana. Though the creative genius of the iPhone may not be the result of smoking weed, it is without question that Chubby Hubby and Truffle Kerfuffle are.

Music: Bob Marley, Bob Dylan, Zayn Malik, Lady Gaga, and Rihanna are just a few musicians who have spoken publicly about their marijuana use. In 2016 Malik told Charlotte Edwardes of Britain's *ES* magazine that "I find it helps me be creative." (Apparently not so much when it comes to being quoted in print.)

Film: Several prominent creators in the film industry have embraced the stoner lifestyle. Seth Rogen, Woody Harrelson, Kirsten Dunst, and Sarah Silverman have been open about their pot use. In fact, Silverman famously revealed her vape pen during a red-carpet interview before the 2014 Emmy Awards.

Other notable celebrities who have credited their creativity to weed include Bill Maher and Joseph Gordon-Levitt. The latter told radio host Howard Stern in 2013 that he was stoned when he first came up with the idea for his movie *Don Jon* and that "the way I use [pot], I absolutely think it has a positive influence on my creative process." (See page 123 for other famous stoners.)

The Beauty of Cannabis

If you're a devotee of beauty and wellness culture, you've no doubt noticed the emergence of what's known as weed beauty. CBD derived from hemp has become one of the trendiest ingredients in the beauty and wellness industry, which has embraced the natural compound in topical products, like lotions and lip balms, and relaxation products, like bath salts and bath bombs.

It's important to note that these products don't contain THC—the psychoactive agent that makes marijuana illegal in certain states and most of the world—which means you don't need a state-issued medical marijuana card to purchase them. If you walk into your local Walgreens, Sephora, or upscale department store, you're likely to find at least one CBD product on the shelf.

CBD began as a natural or "green" beauty ingredient, but in recent years it's gotten a luxury makeover by niche beauty companies Lord Jones, Cannuka, Vertly, and Khus + Khus, which are entirely dedicated to CBD products. These companies, as well as established beauty conglomerates that have incorporated the ingredient into existing beauty and skincare lines, have made strong claims about CBD's ability to act as a powerful antioxidant and anti-inflammatory agent, making it perfect for customers suffering from skin conditions like acne, psoriasis, and eczema as well as chronic joint and muscle pain caused by endometriosis, autoimmune disorders, and scoliosis. One study showed that CBD can slow visible aging in mice, and other studies have noted the compound's anti-inflammatory properties and ability to inhibit sebum production (a cause of acne). However, research is still ongoing, and there aren't enough vetted studies to anoint CBD as a true miracle ingredient. The U.S. Food and Drug Administration regulates the beauty industry, but the Drug Enforcement Administration regulates cannabis-related products, which means no regulatory body is overseeing the amount of CBD in your mascara. Some companies hoping to benefit from the cultural cache of CBD might be skimpy with the stuff, using it to justify a higher price tag without providing an effective product.

If you're interested in CBD products, it will take a bit of homework and sleuthing to find the right ones for you. The cannabisseur knows to consult with a trusted dermatologist and to buy products from verified stockists—never from third-party marketplaces. Start by experimenting with a balm from a brand that you trust, and always patch-test the product on your skin before committing to full and regular use.

Smoking Herb 101

The oldest and traditional way of getting high from marijuana is by smoking the dried and cured buds (or flowers) of a cannabis plant. The cannabisseur has a variety of options for how to smoke one's bud of choice, including the following.

JOINT

The classic never goes out of style. Rolling weed in rolling papers is a nice start, but feel free to expand your options depending on the situation. A pinner is great for just you and a loved one on the beach, whereas rolling a cone is nice for some preconcert festivities. Enjoy a blunt when the guys come over to watch football on Sunday. Or challenge yourself to be the hero of the party by crafting a hand-rolled cross joint with three smoking ends. (This style of joint was made famous in the 2008 movie *Pineapple Express*, starring Seth Rogen and James Franco. It's difficult to master, but if you accomplish it, you and your friends will be truly blessed.)

Pros: Adaptable, affordable, easy to transport

BONG

Water pipes are a cannabisseur must-have.
On the small end of the spectrum, bubblers
are easy to transport and they don't require
the space commitment that comes with a
full-sized bong. That said, a glass bong
is nice to have on hand for special occasions such as 4/20 and Tuesdays. Bongs
can be purchased online or at any local
headshop. (Or make your own; see opposite.)

Pros: Big hits, fun to do with friends

BOWL

Your local specialty store, or head
shop, will have a number of bowl
designs made from wood, plastic, or
glass. Cannabisseurs generally favor glass bowls and
often won't stray from their favorite style. Whatever
you choose, make it uniquely yours and be sure to
keep it safe.

Pros: Compact, easy to use, portable

DIY GRAVITY BONG

For extra-extra-special occasions, when a standard bong just isn't enough, you'll want to explore the gravity bong. This DIY bong is simple to make and extremely effective in its delivery.

First, gather an empty 2-liter bottle, a larger water reservoir such as a bucket, a small piece of foil, and a toothpick. Using scissors or a box cutter, cut off the bottom of the bottle. Fill the large bucket halfway with water. Immerse the cut bottle all the way into the water with the cut side down. Place the foil into the mouthpiece of the bottle, forming a small bowl, and poke tiny holes in it with the toothpick. Pack the bowl with buds from your favorite strain, then light the buds and slowly raise the bottle until it fills with smoke. Don't lift the bottom of the bottle above the surface of the water or the smoke will escape. When the bottle is filled with smoke, remove the bowl, cover the opening with your mouth, and inhale the smoke while pushing down on the bottle. If performed properly, you may begin to question the existence of gravity.

Pros: Bigger hits, even more fun with friends

APPLE

When you're in a pinch and have nothing to smoke out of, pull open the crisper drawer and grab yourself an apple. To make this disposable bowl, you'll need a knife and a pen from which the ink cartridge has been removed. Use the knife to remove the apple's stem, and then burrow the pen halfway into the center of the fruit, where the stem had been. The hole that is created is the main chamber. From one side of the apple, burrow a second hole to meet the main chamber. Finally, burrow a third hole into the side opposite the second hole, again meeting the main chamber. The third hole acts as your shotgun. Dig out a space in the top of the apple to fill with your favorite buds. Once it's packed, light the weed, hold your finger over the shotgun hole, and breathe in through the opposite hole. Who knew fruit could be so much fun?

Pros: Inconspicuous, affordable

SODA CAN

This is the least desirable method for smoking marijuana. That said, it's easy and affordable to make—no specialized equipment necessary—and will give you a certain "street vagrant" feel while you get stoned (especially if you enjoy it along with a bottle of wine tucked in a brown paper bag). First, squeeze an empty soda can in the middle to create a flat sur-

face along one side. Use a small blade to poke several holes in the middle of the flattened side, which will be used to hold your herb. Remove the tab from the can and poke one large hole somewhere in the top that is easy to cover with a finger; this will be your shotgun. Holding the can sideways, place your bud on top of the small holes, hold your finger over the shotgun, and place your mouth over the soda can opening. Light and enjoy.

Pros: Honestly, not many. You're smoking out of a soda can, friend. You may have hit rock bottom.

HOOKAH

A favorite smoking apparatus widely used in the Middle East, India, and Southeast Asia, the hookah has become popular in the U.S. and other countries. It is essentially a water pipe, often fitted with multi-ple tubes that make it ideal for group use. Hookahs can be purchased online, in tobacco shops, or at a local head shop with a large product assortment.

Pros: Great for sharing with a crowd

ONE-HITTER

This underrated method of smoking marijuana generally has the design of a small cigarette, making it easy to travel with, and may be made of glass, metal, or ceramic. To use, press one end of the piece into a "dugout," which is basically a box filled with ground weed packed tightly into one end. Then light and smoke. One-hitters can be purchased online or at most head shops.

Pros: Portable, easy to use

All about Edibles

Whether to protect their lungs, avoid exacerbating respiratory issues, or be discreet, some folks prefer not to smoke. But you can still enjoy a good high with edibles, the general term for any food or drink that is made with concentrated THC. Rather than entering the blood stream through the lungs, as happens when smoking marijuana, the THC in edibles is processed by the stomach and then the liver. As with alcohol, how the substance affects you depends on the amount of food in your stomach and, more specifically, the fat content of that food.

Personal tolerance and dosage also play a role in how an edible affects you; a standard dosage is 10 milligrams THC per serving, but first-time users should start with a half or quarter serving.

The effects of edibles take longer to kick in than when smoking, but they can also be far more potent and longer lasting. So resist the urge to keep nibbling on that brownie until you start to feel its effects—by that time you might have consumed far more THC than you're comfortable with. Always start with small doses of edibles and gradually build up over time until you achieve the desired effect. This will take a process of trial and error (though hopefully not much error), but what a delicious process it will be.

HOMEMADE

Nothing beats a delicious home-baked treat, especially one that can get *you* properly baked as well. Once you master the art of making cannabis-infused oil, the sky is the limit on what you can whip up. Any recipe that calls for oil or butter can be made with the substitution of cannabis oil. (See page 93 for how to make cannabis oil and page 98 for recipes.)

DRINKS

Many companies are now producing and selling THC-infused beverages such as tea, hot chocolate, and even those prepackaged coffee pods. Go slow with drinks—their effects can take even longer than other edibles to set in.

CANDY

Gummy bears, gummy rings, chocolates, caramels—if it's sweet and delicious, there's a good chance you can buy a version of it made with THC oil. Edibles from reputable dispensaries tend to be more consistent in their potency than those acquired by other means. Edible candies purchased on the black market or even those made at home can vary greatly in THC content. The cannabisseur knows that when you find the right candy and the right dosage, you should keep a steady supply on hand.

Cannabis Concentrates

Oils, wax, shatter, and other concentrates are created when THC is extracted from the cannabis plant using a combination of heat, pressure, and solvents. And as with edibles, their effects on the user are more powerful than marijuana that is smoked, so remember to start small and work up to learn your personal tolerance. Because of their unique properties and potency, they cannot always be enjoyed via traditional smoking. Try one of the following methods instead.

VAPING

Originally an alternative to smoking tobacco, vaporizers can be used with THC oil and wax. More commonly referred to as vape pens, they are popular because they emit a vapor (rather than smoke), are odorless, and are easy to transport and use. A typical vape pen operates on a rechargeable battery that connects to a refillable or single-use cartridge filled with THC oil. A small heating unit inside the device called an atomizer is triggered by the user inhaling or by the press of a button. The atomizer heats the oil to nearly 400 degrees Fahrenheit in about 1 second. Because there is no combustion, the key element to creating smoke, what you see in the air as you exhale is the gaseous version of the concentrate.

Heating to a high temperature without burning is the key difference between smoking and vaping.

The cannabisseur always keeps in mind that a vape pen uses a lithium battery and should not be packed inside checked luggage at the airport.

COMBINING WITH HERB

Some concentrates such as wax, hash, and kief can be a great addition to a joint or bowl. Because the potency of these concentrates is higher than that of herb, adding a small amount can go a long way. Try sprinkling kief on the outside of your joint or adding a little wax in your bowl for an extra kick.

DABBING

Dabbing is a method of vaporizing concentrates that might be easily understood as a vape bong. The bong in this case is known as a dab rig, a modified water pipe that can be found in some specialty stores. In the dab rig, a component called the nail is heated with a small torch until it is red-hot and then allowed to briefly cool. A tiny amount ("dab") of concentrate is placed on the nail, which heats it to an extremely high temperature and produces a large amount of vapor that can be inhaled. Shatter is a popular concentrate to use with dabbing that can contain as much as 90 percent THC.

Setting up a rig and mastering the dabbing process is best learned directly from an experienced practitioner, so seek out a staff member at your local head shop who can advise you on the exact equipment and best practices for enjoying concentrates via this method.

Important note: Never use alcohol-based concentrates with dabbing. These are highly combustible and are extremely dangerous to have near a flame, which is a critical element in the dabbing process. If you're curious about dabbing, be sure to learn about the risks and essential safety measures from someone who has first-hand experience.

Legalization of Cannabis

Attitudes about marijuana use are constantly changing, and so are the legal classifications of the drug around the world. It's important to understand the variety of designations and how each affects cultivation, possession, consumption, and distribution. Not to mention that if you travel frequently, the rules at home may not be the same in the country, or even nearby state, you are visiting.

One could argue that legalization offers several advantages (see page 67 for a few). But until use is permitted far and wide, keep in mind these levels of prohibition.

LEGAL FOR RECREATIONAL USE

Legal recreational use is similar to the legality of alcohol consumption—it is permitted under the law and subject to restrictions to ensure safe use. Few countries have legalized the recreational use of marijuana. Notable exceptions include Uruguay, Canada, and some U.S. states (although it is still illegal at the federal level).

LEGAL FOR MEDICAL USE

Some places have laws that treat marijuana as a prescribed drug. Areas that have enacted this approach still have guidelines for how it can be purchased and consumed. Germany, Italy, Israel, the UK, and some U.S. states have legalized a variety of medical uses for marijuana.

ILLEGAL, BUT NOT ENFORCED

Some countries whose laws state that marijuana use is illegal turn a blind eye toward personal consumption of the drug. For example, Bangladesh, Cambodia, Egypt, and India have laws prohibiting recreational use, but these laws are rarely enforced. In places where weed is illegal but usage is not enforced, note that no specific amount of the drug is permitted (unlike in places that have decriminalized it; see below). Visitors should exercise caution.

ILLEGAL

In many countries, the consumption, distribution, possession, and cultivation of marijuana are illegal. In some cases these offenses are punishable by imprisonment for several years—or worse. In Malaysia, for example, an individual arrested and convicted of possessing more than seven ounces of marijuana could be sentenced to death.

DECRIMINALIZATION

An alternative to legalization is decriminalization, which is the process of reducing the severity of punishment for possessing small amounts of marijuana for personal use (amounts vary by location). For example, in 2017 New Hampshire lowered the fine for possession of up to three-quarters of an ounce of marijuana from $1,000 to $200. Other places that have decriminalized have shortened or eliminated prison sentences as punishment for marijuana possession.

Marijuana laws around the world are constantly changing. Make sure to familiarize yourself with local laws before consuming or possessing marijuana while visiting any city. (See also page 122.) Getting high is nice, but not going to prison is way better.

BENEFITS OF LEGALIZATION

In the United States, states where marijuana has been legalized have seen several benefits, namely

Jobs. State legal changes have spawned a booming industry of cannabis companies, including retail stores known as dispensaries, cannabis-based medical product companies, nurseries, and others. Some studies have shown that legalization at the federal level could create more than one million jobs throughout the country.

Economic benefits. Since legalizing marijuana, Washington State, California, and Colorado have seen huge tax revenue increases as a result of marijuana sales. At the current rate of legalization, revenues from marijuana sales in North America are projected to exceed $20 billion by 2021. In addition, legalization reduces the costs associated with drug enforcement and incarceration.

Decreased reliance on the black market. Customers who can legally buy regulated products from licensed dispensaries have less incentive to purchase marijuana from disreputable suppliers with possible ties to drug cartels and organized crime.

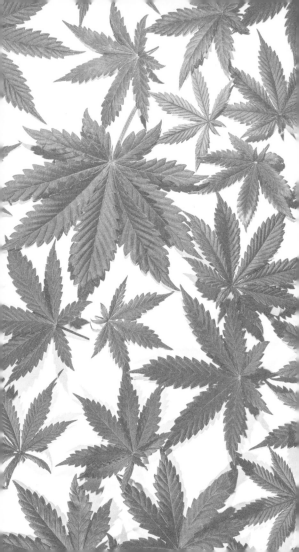

Getting

High

A Crash Course in Cannabisseur Etiquette

Newcomers to the world of cannabis may find it tricky to navigate certain situations. Although the world of marijuana is relaxed and welcoming, and the vast majority of cannabis users will be patient and understanding, it's always wise to familiarize yourself with basic etiquette for several common cannabis-related situations. Read up on the following tips, and remember: you're not eating dinner with the royal family here, so try to enjoy the experience.

PASSING A JOINT

As we learned from the character Smokey in the movie *Friday*, the protocol for sharing a joint with others is "puff, puff, pass." In other words, you may take two drags from the joint before handing it to the person on your left. Avoid holding the joint for too long, allowing it to burn needlessly, and moistening the end with your saliva. This last faux pas is known as *lipping* a joint, and nothing advertises "rookie" more than that. Saying thank you to the person who supplied the joint is nice but not necessary. The best way to express your gratitude is to bring your own joint to share the next time.

BYOB

That's Bring Your Own Bud. If you know that you'll be attending a gathering where people will be smoking weed, it is always good form to bring some of your own—for example, preground buds, a vape pen, or even a joint to pass. (Don't stress if you forgot; people will figure that you were probably just high.)

SHOPPING AT DISPENSARIES

Dispensaries in the United States are a relatively new phenomenon. Other than being polite and friendly with your budtender, the main thing to know is that they won't accept a credit card and you must pay with cash (see page 91 for more on navigating your local dispensary). Asking questions is good; dispensary employees usually like to show off their knowledge.

SHOPPING AT HEAD SHOPS

These specialty stores carry most any type of weed paraphernalia you might need. Everything from bowls and bongs to grinders and vaporizers are available for purchase. Although the employees at these stores under-stand what the likely use will be of these products, in places where recreational marijuana use is illegal you should exercise discretion. Don't mention anything about marijuana, and avoid using the terms *bowl* and *bong.* Instead, refer to the weed as *flowers,* or mention tobacco, and use the terms *pipe* or *water pipe.* Some head shops display signage about this etiquette to remind you, but follow this practice even if they don't.

ATTENDING A WEED PARTY

If you are invited to a weed party, odds are that you're already familiar with the proper etiquette. Regardless, remember to bring some form of marijuana, your favorite munchies if appropriate, and a positive attitude. The keys to any successful weed party are the people and the environment, so have fun. (Want to throw a weed party of your own? See page 108.)

NAVIGATING A MIXED CROWD

Suppose you find yourself at a party or other social gathering where some people are enjoying a smoke and others are not. Although smoking marijuana has become more socially acceptable, it is still illegal in most places and can be met with a variety of attitudes and opinions. If you are comfortable with joining in, don't be shy. Weed smokers are generally a friendly bunch. Depending on how familiar you are with the folks in attendance (both smokers and abstainers), you may want to avoid overdoing it. If you're concerned about becoming preoccupied with how you are perceived by nonsmokers at the party, consider sitting this one out. Otherwise, embrace that which makes you happy. Perhaps those who aren't participating today will partake on another day.

Equipment Every Cannabisseur Should Own

As a cannabisseur, you don't have to stock up on all sorts of fancy gadgets and gear, but a few key items will help you maximize your experience and enjoyment—in addition to this book, of course. (Seriously, if you are reading this at a friend's house or in a store, get your own copy. And you call yourself a cannabisseur?)

FIRE

You can never have too many lighters on hand. After all, weed doesn't smoke itself, right? Keep it simple. The basic convenience-store lighter does the job; avoid butane lighters or Zippos. Keeping track of your light can become tougher with every use, so don't invest in anything fancy.

BOWL

There are literally thousands of bowls out there in assorted materials, shapes, and designs. The cannabisseur takes time with this purchase to find the bowl that best fits their personality and smoking needs. For some, the ideal bowl is one they've had since college, or that they found at a favorite concert—one that seems to hit just right and adds a certain nostalgic quality to every use. Others want a fancy one-of-a-kind design. The right bowl can last years, if not decades, and is likely to be used countless times, so choose carefully and do your best to keep it safe from breaking.

ONE-HITTER

The one-hitter, which can be purchased as a set with a dugout, is a must-have. Because its design often mimics that of a cigarette, smoking from it can be more discreet compared to other options. Ground weed that has been packed into the dugout in advance makes using it quick and easy—all you do is smush (technical term) the one-hitter into the ground weed, light, and smoke.

VAPE PEN

Vape pens are available in many different sizes and can be used with either plant material or concentrates (see page 61 for more). The cannabisseur may own several, but an oil pen is truly essential. It requires no advance preparation, making it great when you are on the go. It's also ideal when you don't want the smoke and odor of traditional herb smoking.

GRINDER

Grinders are used to break apart marijuana buds into very small pieces. They can be metal or plastic, are available in various sizes, and often come in fun colors and designs. Grinders play a critical role in best preparing the buds for smoking out of bowls, bongs, or one-hitters, but they are also essential for use in rolling great joints. The best grinder is likely made of metal, will be extremely durable, and should contain a filter for extracting kief from ground buds. (Kief is the high-potency resinous material that coats the marijuana buds, and having a filter in your grinder will allow you to add a little kick when it is sprinkled on top of a packed bowl, inside or outside of a rolled joint, or mixed into ground weed.) You can legally purchase grinders online or at specialty/head shops.

ROLLING PAPERS

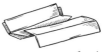

The fine art of joint rolling may be lost on some, but the canna-bisseur knows that old school never goes out of style when it comes to marijuana use. Always have rolling papers on hand, and remember that you have several purchasing options. For single use or sharing with a few people, 1¼-inch papers should do the trick. If you tend to pass joints around in groups, have a supply of 1½-inch or double-wide rolling papers for larger joints and easier cone rolling. (Speaking of cones, prerolled cones are available online or at head shops and can be a great time-saver. Simply fill them tightly with ground weed, twist the end, smoke, and enjoy.)

Are Smell-Proof Bags Worth It?

Smell-proof bags are available online and will effectively contain the scent of your buds. These are great for traveling when you don't want the strong smell to attract attention, but they are not recommended as a storage option. To best maintain the freshness and potency of your flowers, there is no substitute for a mason jar. For more tips on storage, see page 89.

How to Roll a Joint

Smoking a joint is a simple, timeless pleasure and an ideal way to appreciate the subtle characteristics of the marijuana flower. Knowing how to roll your own enhances the experience.

This essential cannabisseur skill may seem easy to learn but in fact it can take a lifetime to master. These steps will set you up for success. Variations follow.

What you need:

- Marijuana
- Rolling papers (1¼ inch for a small group, or double-wide for a crowd)
- Filter (optional)
- Grinder (optional)
- Pen cap
- Lighter

1. **Prepare the mix.** Carefully sift through your marijuana buds of choice with your fingers to remove unwanted lumps, seeds, or stems. If desired, grind the buds with a grinder to help ensure an even consistency.

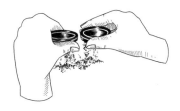

2. **Insert a filter.** Lay the rolling paper flat on a surface, with the sticky-tab side up. Place the filter on one end of the rolling paper along the center fold. If you don't have a filter, you can tear a piece of cardboard off the rolling paper case and roll it into a cylinder.

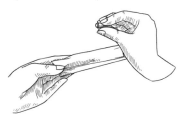

3. **Fill the rolling paper.** Fill the paper with the marijuana mix and spread the mix evenly down the fold—but not on top of the filter. Try to avoid a pile-up in the middle. The mix should be about cigarette height.

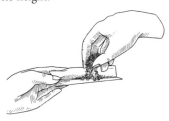

4. **Shape the joint.** Pinch the paper near the ends. Slowly roll it back and forth. Move your fingers across the joint as you work to maintain a cylindrical shape.

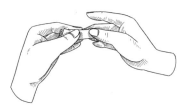

5. **Roll the joint.** Fold the side of the paper without the sticky tab into the joint. Roll the joint with your thumbs, moving toward the sticky tab. Try to keep the roll tight.

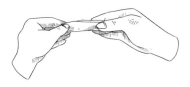

6. **Seal the joint.** As you approach the top of the rolling paper, lick the sticky tab. Roll the joint up through the sticky tab to seal it along the outer seam.

7. **Pack the joint.** You should have an evenly rolled cylinder with an open edge at the top and the filter at the bottom. Use a pen cap to push the marijuana down from the open edge to pack it tightly.

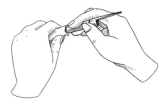

8. **Twist, light, and smoke.** Once you have tamped the marijuana down into the joint, twist the top closed. Light the twisted end. Enjoy!

Variations: To roll a **cone**, use a double-wide rolling paper and follow steps 1 and 2 as above. In step 3, sprinkle a small amount of the mix at one end of the rolling paper and increase the amount as you move to the opposite end. One end should be fuller than the other, creating the desired cone shape. Proceed with steps 4 through 6. After tamping down the mix in step 7, you may wish to add more of the mix to fill the cone. Then twist, light, and smoke.

To roll a **blunt** or **cone blunt**, substitute a cigar wrap for the rolling paper. Proceed with directions as above.

How to Do a Bong Hit

Bongs, aka water pipes, are completely legal and may be purchased in most head shops. They are not intended to be sold for use with marijuana (unless it is legal in that particular state), so be sure not to reference marijuana when making your purchase. Bongs can vary in shape, size, and material, but the majority will work with the following instructions.

Note: True cannabisseurs own only glass bongs; plastic won't cut it. Staffers at head shops are generally very friendly and eager to assist you with your purchase, so be sure to ask questions to help you make the right purchase.

What you need:

- Marijuana
- Grinder (optional)
- Bong
- Water
- Ice cubes (optional)
- Lighter

1. Remove the bowl-and-stem portion of the bong, and pack it tightly with your preferred choice of marijuana. Grinding your weed first is optional but preferred since it will provide a more consistent hit. Set aside the packed bowl.

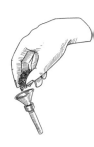

2. Fill the base of your bong with water (preferably ice cold). The water level should be high enough to cover the bottom of the stem when it is inserted, but not so high that water can get into the stem and wet your buds.

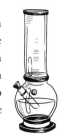

3. Add ice cubes, if desired, to the main tube of the bong. This will create a colder, smoother hit and may reduce coughing.

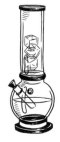

4. Insert the packed bowl into the bong. Place your mouth tightly against the inside of the opening of the tube and hold a flame gently over the bowl, allowing the weed to burn. Gently inhale as the water bubbles and smoke begins to fill the chamber.

Tip: Start slow, allowing only a small amount of smoke to accumulate in the chamber before you remove the flame and stop inhaling.

5. Once your desired amount of smoke is in the chamber, remove the flame, carefully pull the bowl out of the chamber, and take a breath of fresh air.

6. With the bowl removed and smoke in the chamber, inhale all of the smoke (aka "pull" the smoke) from the chamber. Hold the smoke in your lungs for a few seconds, and then exhale fully.

How to Grow Cannabis Indoors

If you are serious about planning your own "grow," it's recommended that you consult additional resources. Entire books are dedicated to the subject, and websites such as Leafly.com offer a wealth of information too. Be sure to consider the following factors before jumping into the world of marijuana production.

Decide on the number of plants. As a beginner, start with one or two, which will be easier to monitor than a whole crop. Should things go awry, the mistakes will be less costly as well.

Identify a "grow room." Good options include a closet, cabinet, or spare bedroom. Be sure to identify a space that will accommodate the number of plants, their eventual growth height (some varieties can grow as tall as 13 feet), and the equipment necessary for them to flourish. The ideal space is convenient for you to access, sanitized and easy to clean, completely closed off from sunlight, cool and dry with access to fresh air, and concealed from unwanted attention (think nosy neighbors or disapproving family members).

Stock up on essentials. For a proper grow, you'll need to invest in the following materials and equipment:

- **Seeds:** Select seeds based on your personal preference. See page 31 for a discussion of the type of strains and their individual characteristics.

- **Prefertilized organic soil:** Cannabis plants require a variety of nutrients including nitrogen, phosphorus, potassium, calcium, magnesium, iron, and copper. This type of soil is recommended for beginner growers.

- **Lighting:** Experts say that lighting is the most critical external factor affecting the quality and quantity of your grow. Research lighting set-ups to identify which option will work best for your strain and allocated space. Top choices are HID (high intensity discharge), fluorescent, and LED grow lights. Your plants will require 18 hours of light and 6 hours of darkness.

- **Fans and filters:** Access to fresh air is essential for the photosynthesis process. Your grow room will need vents, fans, and filters to keep air circulating.

- **Automation equipment:** You'll want to set monitors to control lighting, temperature and humidity. As a beginner, use a programmable thermostat for best results.

Choose your grow method. The two most popular methods for growing cannabis indoors are in soil and hydroponically. High-quality, organic prefertilized soil is best for beginners, requiring a simple plant pot that allows water to drain through the bottom. The hydroponic method, which helps plants grow faster but requires more precision, feeds the nutrients directly into the roots through osmosis. You can find tutorials online when you're ready to take your grow to the next level.

Be patient. After the initial set-up, check growth daily and be prepared to wait. Even when you automate parts of the growing process, cannabis plants may take several months to develop buds that are ready to be harvested (see page 27 for more information on the phases of growth and harvesting).

How to Store Your Pot

A perfectly cured bud can last up to two years under ideal conditions. Improperly stored weed can lose potency and cannabinoid content. Maximize the potency and shelf life of your marijuana with these tips.

STORAGE DOS

- Keep your marijuana in an airtight glass mason jar. These are available online, at craft stores, or anywhere that sells kitchen supplies.

- Store your mason jar in a cool and dark place. Avoid sunlight and keep your jar in an environment that has a temperature below 75 degrees. Stoves or other heat sources are your herb's enemy.

- If you are a cigar aficionado or just have some spare cash, buy yourself a humidor. Marijuana is best kept at a relative humidity of 54 to 63 percent.

- As an alternative or in addition to a humidor, you can control the humidity of your storage space with Boveda packs. These reusable pouches are similar to those little silica gel packets you find packed in new shoes; they contain water-absorbent beads and salts that help maintain a specific level of relative humidity. You can tuck them directly into the mason jar, along with your weed. Find them online or at specialty head shops.

STORAGE DON'TS

- Don't store marijuana in aluminum foil or plastic zip-top bags; without an airtight seal, it will dry out quickly.

- Don't freeze your green or keep it in extremely low temperatures. Although there's debate about whether this causes damage, why risk it?

- Avoid handling weed roughly or more than is necessary. Preserving the original form of your buds will help keep them fresh longer. Be nice to your weed and it will be nice to you!

How to Navigate a Dispensary

Some U.S. states have legalized the recreational use of marijuana and have made it available for sale in specialized stores known as dispensaries. Dispensaries can vary dramatically in the products they offer and the quality of service they provide. Here's what you need to know before walking into one for the first time.

Bring cash. Despite that marijuana is legal in some states, it is still classified at the federal level as a Schedule I substance. This means that federally regulated banks cannot legally support marijuana dispensaries, so these operations are cash only.

Know your desired effect. Much like walking into a bar, the employee at a dispensary will ask you what you would like. This is your opportunity to describe what you want to get out of your marijuana experience so that they can recommend products that make the most sense for you. Some folks are looking for a product to enjoy while being enveloped by their sofa and marveling at the size of the universe. Others may want something they can enjoy during a night out with friends at a club. Whatever your desired effect, most dispensaries have options for you to choose from.

Don't be shy. Feel free to use your time with a dispensary staff member to ask questions about possible purchases. You may want to know what the proper dosage of an edible is for you or how long you can expect a high to last. No matter the question, most employees are happy to spend the time answering questions and explaining products in detail.

Try something new. The options for marijuana consumption in a dispensary can be overwhelming, and there will surely be items that you've never seen before. Now is a perfect opportunity to try cannabis-infused hot chocolate or tea, lotions, candies, and prerolled joints. Variety is one of the great advantages to legalized marijuana sales, so be sure to take advantage on your dispensary adventure.

Cooking with Cannabis

Love to eat? Love to get high? Why not combine these two pastimes? Before you can start cooking up your first batch of marijuana-laced brownies, you have to make cannabis oil, the required ingredient for most any delicious edible treat. Because THC, the psychoactive component in marijuana, is fat soluble, edible oils are an ideal way to incorporate it into recipes. Here's how to make a batch of your own.

1. **Grind and decarb your weed.** The term *decarb* refers to decarboxylation, which is the process that maximizes marijuana's psychoactive and relaxing effects. Usually, this occurs when you smoke it, but in the case of edibles you can decarb weed by baking it.

    Preheat your oven to 200 degrees Fahrenheit. In a high-powered kitchen blender, grind weed to your desired consistency. (Only grind and decarb as much as you intend to use right away.) Line a baking sheet or toaster tray with a sheet of parchment paper, and spread the ground weed evenly on the tray. Bake for 75 minutes.

2. **Choose your base oil.** Vegetable oil is the most versatile option—you can use it for most any recipe, savory or sweet. But other neutral oils like coconut, canola, or grapeseed will work as well.

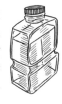

3. **Choose your cooking apparatus.** The process will take several hours (see Note on page 96), so cooking options include a slow cooker, double-boiler, or saucepan. My preference is a slow cooker because it reduces smell and allows you to maintain a consistent temperature for an extended period.

4. **Mix your ingredients.** The following amounts are my preferred portions, but you may want more or less marijuana. Do what is best for you. Just keep in mind that every quarter ounce of weed used in baking yields approximately 700 milligrams of THC in your edibles. (This is based on a strain with 10 percent THC content; your strain may vary.)

To make approximately 1 cup of cannabis oil, mix together in a bowl:

- 1¼ cups of vegetable or other base oil

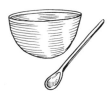

- ½ ounce of ground and decarbed marijuana buds

- 4 cups of water

- 2 teaspoons of lecithin powder (see Note, below)

Note: Lecithin powder is a supplement sold at most pharmacies and vitamin stores. In cannabis oil it acts as a booster, ensuring that your edibles high hits quicker and lasts longer. A little goes a long way—add just 1 teaspoon per quarter ounce of weed.

5. **Cook.** Add oil mixture to the slow cooker and cook on low for 4 to 8 hours. We suggest stirring gently every 30 minutes, but it's not essential.

Note: Though edible oils can be made in less than an hour, the longer you let the THC infuse into your base oil, the more potent it will be. More powerful cannabis oil means you can make a larger or a stronger batch of edibles, depending on your taste. Consider allowing as much as 8 hours of cooking time for best results. (Some chefs will cook it longer, but I have seen no significant difference in quality or potency beyond 8 hours.)

6. **Drain and strain.** Line an ordinary kitchen strainer with cheesecloth and place a strainer over a large pot or bowl. Strain the cooked liquid. I recommend straining the mixture a second time, using a double thickness of cheesecloth. This will minimize any sediment in the oil, which may affect the taste of your edibles. **Important note:** Save your strained weed! Chances are you probably did not extract all the THC, so save it, freeze it, and add to your next batch of cannabis oil for an extra kick.

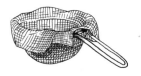

Your finished product may be a shade of green or even yellow, and it may not look the same every time you make it. Don't worry; this has nothing to do with potency and is often a by-product of the particular strain of marijuana used.

Substitute cannabis oil for cooking oil in your favorite recipe and voilà! You'll have yourself a delicious treat that will also get you high. Infused canola oil can last for up to 2 years; store in the freezer until ready for use.

For even more kitchen inspiration, see the recipes beginning on page 98.

5 Cannabis Recipes for Any and All Occasions

Although you can modify any of your favorite recipes to be made with cannabis oil, here are a few simple but delicious ideas to get you started. Before you begin the following recipes, be sure to infuse your oil first (see page 93) because this step takes the most time. The servings indicated for each recipe include approximately 10 to 20 milligrams THC each; remember that if you're new to edibles, you'll want to start with smaller portions.

INFUSED-CHOCOLATE-DIPPED STRAWBERRIES
Serves 4

Ingredients

    2 tablespoons of cannabis-infused
       coconut oil
    1½ cups of chocolate chips
    12 large strawberries (with stems)

Directions

In a medium microwave-safe bowl, stir together the infused oil and chocolate chips. Microwave on high power for 30 seconds. Remove and stir.

Continue to microwave in 15-second intervals, stirring after each, until chocolate is completely melted. Then let cool to room temperature.

Line a baking sheet with parchment paper. Dip the strawberries into the melted chocolate. Set on the prepared sheet and refrigerate, uncovered, for about 30 minutes or until the chocolate is firm.

INFUSED CRISP RICE SQUARES
Serves 4 to 6

Ingredients
¼ cup of cannabis-infused coconut oil
1 10.5-ounce bag of marshmallows
5 cups of crisp rice cereal

Directions
Line a 9-inch square baking pan with foil and spray foil with nonstick cooking spray. Set aside.

In a large saucepan over medium heat, combine the infused oil and marshmallows and stir constantly until completely melted, about 4 to 5 minutes. Keep stirring so that the bottom doesn't burn.

Once mixture is smooth, reduce heat to low, add cereal, and mix until cereal is evenly coated.

Pour into the prepared pan, pressing into place with a spoon, and let cool for about an hour. Cut into squares and serve.

Variation: For less potent treats, use 2 tablespoons of infused oil and 2 tablespoons of regular coconut oil.

INFUSED BROWNIES
Serves 8 to 10

Ingredients

2 large eggs, lightly beaten
⅓ cup of water
⅓ cup of cannabis-infused oil
1 box of store-bought brownie mix
    (enough for a 9-by-13-inch pan)
½ cup of lightly sweetened chocolate chips
¼ cup of crushed pecans

Directions

Preheat the oven to 330 degrees Fahrenheit. Grease a 9-by-13-inch baking pan with butter or cooking spray. Set aside.

In a large mixing bowl, stir together the eggs, water, and infused oil. Stir in the brownie mix, chocolate chips, and pecans until mixture is uniform. Pour the batter into the prepared pan.

Bake according to the package instructions or for about 30 minutes. Brownies are done when a toothpick inserted into the center comes out clean.

Remove the pan from the oven and allow to cool to room temperature. Cut brownies into squares and serve.

SPAGHETTI BOLO-HAZE
Serves 4

Ingredients

2–3 tablespoons of cannabis-infused olive oil
    (depending on desired strength), divided
1 pound of ground beef
Salt and pepper, to taste
1 onion, diced
2 large carrots, diced
2 celery stalks, diced
2 garlic cloves, chopped
¼ cup red wine
2 tablespoons of tomato paste
1 28-ounce can of crushed tomatoes
2 cups of beef stock
1 16-ounce package of dried spaghetti

Directions

In a large saucepan over medium-high heat, warm
about half of the infused oil. Add the ground beef
with a pinch of salt and pepper. Cook the beef until
well browned, then transfer to a bowl and set aside.

Add the remaining infused oil to the same saucepan and warm over medium heat. Add the onions,
carrots, and celery. Cook and gently stir for about 5

minutes, until onions are just translucent. Season with salt and pepper to taste. Add the garlic and cook for an additional 2 minutes. Add the ground beef back into the saucepan, along with any oil that has accumulated in the bowl.

Turn the heat to high. Add wine and tomato paste and gently stir, scraping up any stuck-on bits from the bottom of the pan, until the liquid has reduced to a sticky glaze.

Add crushed tomatoes to the saucepan and stir well. Pour in the beef stock, reduce the heat to low, and simmer for about 40 minutes or until the sauce is thickened, stirring occasionally.

While the sauce simmers, bring a large pot of heavily salted water to a rapid boil. Cook the spaghetti according to the package instructions until al dente. Reserve some of the pasta water, then drain the pasta, adding it to your bolo-haze sauce. Stir to incorporate. If the sauce is too thick, add about ¼ cup of the reserved pasta water to thin it out. Mix well and serve warm.

INFUSED BANANA PANCAKES
Serves 6

Ingredients

    1 cup of all-purpose flour

    1 tablespoon of granulated sugar

    2 teaspoons of baking powder

    ¼ teaspoon of salt

    2 tablespoons of cannabis-infused vegetable oil

    1 egg, lightly beaten

    1 cup of milk

    2 ripe bananas, mashed

Directions

In a small bowl, combine the flour, sugar, baking powder, and salt.

In another bowl, mix together the infused oil, egg, milk, and mashed bananas.

Slowly stir the flour mixture into the banana mixture until incorporated. The batter will be lumpy.

Heat a lightly oiled griddle or frying pan over medium-high heat. (Feel free to use a little more infused oil to coat the pan if you'd like.) For each pancake, pour ¼ cup of batter onto the hot pan and cook until bubbles start to form. Flip and cook until golden brown on both sides. Serve and enjoy.

Variation: Substitute infused coconut oil one-for-one for the vegetable oil to give these pancakes a subtly sweeter, slightly tropical flavor.

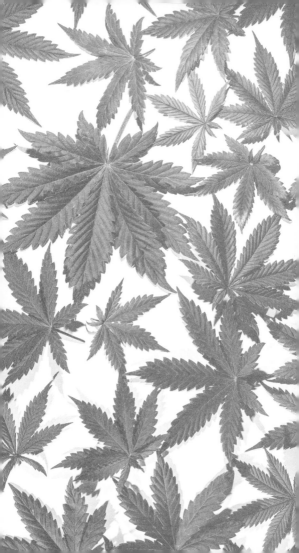

Living
Your Best
Cannabisseur
Life

How to Throw a Weed Party

In recent years, as marijuana use has become more prevalent, people have found ways to create social events devoted to it. These get-togethers are often centered on a particular holiday and present an opportunity to try various cannabis products as well as new methods for consuming them.

Weed parties likely stem from the tradition of people getting together each year on the twentieth of April to get high with friends. These gatherings, which were a kind of underground celebration of all things cannabis, became known as "420 parties." The number 420 is believed by some to be the police code for "marijuana smoking in progress" in the 1970s (see page 120 for the real story), and it is still a common reference used today.

But weed parties have evolved significantly to match the endless creativity from those who throw them. Of course, the marijuana doesn't hurt with those creative juices either. Some of the best theme ideas include Hallo-weed, Danksgiving, Chronica, and New Year's Tokin' Eve. But celebrations of more obscure holidays work too, such as Hash Wednesday, Joint Pass-over, Roach Hash-anah, and Arbor Day (it's a day to celebrate plants, don't overthink it).

Whatever occasion you are celebrating with a weed party, find ways to make your fete unique. Ask attendees to bring their favorite strains of cannabis and their favorite munchies to share. Offer different consumption methods in various rooms—think edibles in the kitchen, bong hits in the basement, and vaping in the living room. For parties held on a traditional gift-giving holiday, try a white elephant exchange or perhaps the infamous Saran Wrap Ball Party Game (see page 110 for instructions).

THE SARAN WRAP BALL PARTY GAME

Buy yourself the biggest box of plastic wrap you can find, along with prizes for players to win. These might include candy, lottery tickets, joints, or any fun gag gift that your friends will enjoy.

Start by wrapping the largest prize in plastic wrap and continue to wrap until it is mostly covered. Add prizes as you keep wrapping around the center item. It is important to wrap in all directions to create the shape of a ball. A successful ball should include plenty of prizes and be big enough to wow your guests. If you have a large number of people attending, consider wrapping two balls to be passed around simultaneously.

Let the games begin! All players form a circle. Select one person to start unwrapping the ball, and have the person immediately to their right roll a pair of dice while the first person unwraps. As soon as the second person rolls doubles, the player unwrapping must stop and pass the ball to the person on their right. If they were able to successfully remove any prizes, they get to keep them. The dice are passed to the right as well, and play continues. The game ends when all prizes have been unwrapped from the ball.

Games to Play with Friends

Getting a group of friends together to blaze some chronic is a perfect opportunity to play a fun game. Keeping it simple is your best bet; the more complicated the game, the more likely you will lose your crowd. Remembering things like rules or whose turn it is when stoned can be a bit . . . complicated. Here are some favorites.

CARDS AGAINST HUMANITY

This game has become an American classic for adults to play when the kids aren't around. They call it a party game for horrible people, and you will quickly learn just how horrible you and your friends really are.

VIDEO GAMES

One- or two-player video games are always fun to play when you're high. Which games are best? Simpler is usually better, and any game in which following the storyline is important should be avoided. Some folks love racing games like *Mario Kart*, *Gran Turismo*, and *Burnout 3: Takedown*. For others, immersion into a different world is best; think *Grand Theft Auto*, *Call of Duty*, and *Fortnite*. Old-school classics like *Super Mario Bros.*, *Contra*, and *Punch-Out!!* are straightforward and will keep you entertained for hours.

BEER PONG

Playing beer pong while stoned can be incredibly satisfying when you find yourself locked in to the target. It can be equally brutal when you realize that you have smoked entirely way too much to play competently. Similar to the effects of alcohol, the right amount of weed can have you in a zone, confident and feeling like you can't miss. But a few too many puffs, and you may let your teammate down in a big way.

DISTURBED FRIENDS

As the name suggests, this card game is a great way to see just how messed up your buddies are. One player reads aloud a multiple-choice question about some incredibly awkward but hilarious scenario, and other players vote on what they think the first player's answer is. It may be the last time you hang out with some of these people after learning what you think about one another, so be sure to enjoy your time together playing this game.

JOKING HAZARD

This game will introduce you to two comic characters known as Cyanide and Happiness. Create a comic storyline for them using cards provided. The scenarios that ensue will leave your face hurting from laughter.

C**KSUCKER

A simple yet somehow complicated DIY game that involves nothing more than you and a few friends sitting in a circle. One person starts by saying the number 1 out loud. The person to their left follows by saying the number 2, and this continues around the circle in the same direction. When the next number in the sequence has a 7 in it (e.g., 7, 17, 27, etc.), is a multiple of 7 (e.g., 14, 21, 28, etc.), or has double digits (e.g., 11, 22, 33, etc.), the player whose turn it is must say "c**ksucker" instead of the number, and then the counting switches to the opposite direction. So if you say the number 6, the person next to you says "c**ksucker" instead of 7, and it is back to you to say 8 and on around the circle until the number 11 comes up. Get to 100 without a slip-up and you are world champions! For a family-friendly variation, try changing the name of this game to Puppydogs.

Satisfying the Munchies

One of the inevitable side effects of enjoying marijuana is an increase in appetite, and often for very specific tastes. This can be very beneficial as a medicinal effect for chemotherapy patients who have difficulty eating or a diminished appetite. For recreational users, this is an opportunity to devour those perfect snacks that take us right to our happy place. Until the next morning, at least, when we hop on the scale.

Although there is still debate on this topic, some studies have shown that THC, the primary active ingredient in marijuana, binds to receptors in the olfactory bulb of the human brain, the region that processes odors. This seems to enhance our sensitivity to smells and tastes, which makes different foods seem more desirable when we're stoned.

Studies have also shown that one effect of THC is an increased release in dopamine, which enhances the pleasure we experience from eating. They have also shown that, like alcohol, marijuana can lower our inhibitions. So even though we know we shouldn't eat that package of raw cookie dough, we may be less inclined to say no to our urge to do so.

Whatever the reason, munchies are a critical part of the marijuana experience, so here are just a few of our absolute favorite ways to satisfy them.

Oreo cookies. Double stuffed are preferable, for reasons that I shouldn't have to explain. But what about triple stuffed, you say? Write your own book, my friend.

Doritos. We won't get into the debate of which flavor is best, because Spicy Nacho reigns over all others. Period.

Pizza. Put whatever you want on it, your pie will undoubtedly be perfect.

Packaged ramen noodles. Warm, hearty, and delicious. Eating them will take you right back to your college days, except that now you can afford way better weed.

Cereal. I'm not talking about bran flakes here, folks. I mean the kind of cereal that makes children cry in the supermarket when they aren't allowed to have it. Cinnamon Toast Crunch, Cocoa Pebbles, peanut butter Cap'n Crunch, and Krave are all highly recommended. You'll thank me later.

How to Deal with a Bad High

Marijuana is a naturally grown drug that has been used for centuries with minimal side effects. That said, most pot smokers will tell you that at some point they have experienced a bad high. It rarely lasts long and generally involves a higher-than-usual level of anxiety or paranoia. To avoid finding yourself in this situation, keep in mind these tips.

Know your limits. Weed consumption is never a contest, and your best bet is to start slow. Remember that you can always smoke more to add to your experience, so try not to overdo it. Edibles in particular should be taken in smaller incremental doses until you know the right amount for you. An edible high lasts longer than one achieved by other means, and potency can vary greatly if the items you're consuming came from a source other than a dispensary.

Relax. Sometimes, no matter where you are or the amount of weed you consume, you just start bugging out a little. The best thing to do in this situation is to breathe in through your nose and out through your mouth. Deep cleansing breaths will help you stay calm and cool.

Positive surroundings, positive experience. If you tend to feel a little paranoid when stoned, downing an infused brownie before boarding a plane or watching a horror movie isn't the smartest idea. A great way to avoid a bad high is to put yourself in a place you *want* to be, such as an intimate gathering with trusted friends or on your comfy couch, watching your favorite show with your main squeeze.

Hydrate. The cannabisseur always has a bottle of water handy, and maybe some Kool-Aid too, if available. A good IPA may be a great way to accentuate your high, but if you're freaking out, reach for water instead.

Find a distraction. Video games, movies, and good friends are all great ways to steer your mind away from thinking that people are staring at you or that the police are monitoring your home. Remember that those things aren't really happening (and if they are, your issues go well beyond how much weed you smoked). Focus on something pleasurable, and this too shall pass.

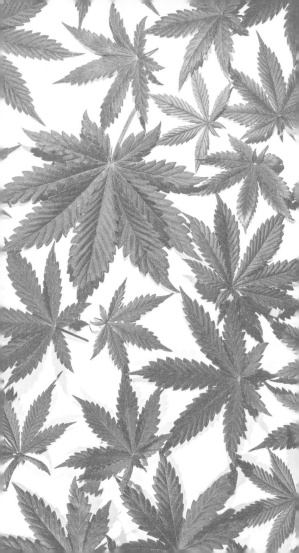

The Culture
of Cannabis

The Cannabisseur's Favorite Holiday: 4/20

If there's one thing every cannabisseur knows, it's that April 20 is an annual holiday devoted to weed, because 420 is the old 1970s police code for "marijuana smoking in progress." Right?

Wrong. And stop being such a know-it-all.

The real story begins in 1971 with a group of five California high school students who called themselves the Waldos. The friends would meet at 4:20 p.m. outside their school to smoke pot and search a nearby forest for an abandoned cannabis plant they had heard about. They even had a treasure map to help them with their search. Unfortunately, they never found the plant, but they did coin a term that will be forever associated with smoking pot. For a while, "420" was a great code for students to use to talk about weed and avoid detection by parents or teachers. Eventually the adults caught on.

And so the legend of 420 was born, and it was only a matter of time before the ritual of lighting up when the clock struck twenty minutes past four gave way to an entire day of the year dedicated to all things cannabis. Indeed, April 20 has become an international holiday among pot smokers and has spawned new and creative ways of celebrating. Some folks attempt challenges such as smoking within 100 feet of a police station, getting someone high for the first time, or creating the greatest snack combination ever. Others mark the occasion by gathering with friends who enjoy weed to share new and favorite strains, sample the latest vape pen, or enjoy homemade edibles. These so-called 4/20 parties have traditionally been kept on the down-low, although now they are becoming more mainstream.

In California, where recreational marijuana use has been legalized, 4/20 events have cropped up all over the state. There is no shortage of festivals, movie screenings, and concerts available to enjoy that day, and dispensaries tend to run special sales around the event. Hippie Hill in San Francisco is not to be missed. Colorado also has an array of events, including the free Mile High 420 Festival in Denver. This is the busiest time of the year for dispensaries there, with people traveling from all over to enjoy the festivities. Vancouver, Amsterdam, Prague, Seattle, and other cities have become popular destinations for 4/20 celebrations, and more are cropping up every year.

If you plan to travel for your 4/20 celebrations, see the Note on the next page to ensure a safe—and prison-free—trip.

Note: When traveling for 4/20, be sure to familiarize yourself and comply with local laws regarding public consumption. For U.S. travel, the National Conference of State Legislatures, which maintains an informative "Marijuana Overview" page on its website (ncsl.org), with up-to-date legalization status in each state. For international travel, Kindland (thekindland.com) and Quartz (qz.com) have published comprehensive global roundups.

But because legality is always changing, a quick internet search may be most accurate for the most current information on your destination of choice. Be safe, and have fun!

Famous Stoners

Marijuana has had a constant presence in the entertainment industry since the early 1900s, when jazz musicians preferred its effect on their creativity and performance stamina, rather than the dulling inebriation of alcohol. Its popularity surged within the music industry when rock icon Bob Dylan introduced pot to the Beatles during their first visit to New York in 1964. In the second half of the twentieth century, pot was a staple of the hippie music of Haight-Ashbury and, later, in Compton's hip-hop scene.

The twenty-first century has seen marijuana proliferate throughout the pop culture universe, with actors, comics, and other entertainers joining musicians in extolling its benefits. Celebrity endorsements, along with increasing legalization of the drug, have helped make it more mainstream in the U.S. and around the world.

Medicinal and recreational pot use in the pop-culture world goes way beyond Willie Nelson and Seth Rogen. Comedian, TV star, and actress Whoopi Goldberg; singer and weed entrepreneur Melissa Etheridge; talk show host Montel Williams; film mega-star Charlize Theron; and even celebrated poet Maya Angelou have publicly discussed their love for marijuana. Following are some of weed culture's greatest icons.

SNOOP DOGG

This iconic rapper, singer, songwriter, music producer, TV star, and entrepreneur is just as known for his weed-loving lifestyle as he is for his career accomplishments. In 2018, Snoop took his love of cannabis to a new level by cofounding the venture capital firm Casa Verde Capital and actively funding up-and-coming cannabis companies, including vaporization hardware businesses and business-to-business marketplaces. In 2007 he discussed his pro-marijuana stance on the Dutch late-night talk show *Jensen!*, saying: "So what if I'm smokin' weed onstage and doing what I gotta do? It's not me shooting nobody, stabbing nobody, killing nobody. It's a peaceful gesture and [critics] have to respect that and appreciate that."

CHEECH AND CHONG

The award-winning comedic duo of Richard Marin and Tommy Chong based their careers of stand-up comedy and cult-classic movies on their enjoyment of weed. Beginning in October 2003, Chong served eight months in jail for conspiring to distribute drug paraphernalia after the federal government raided his "glass" company. In April 2018, on *The Late Show with Stephen Colbert*, the comics expressed displeasure that marijuana was no longer "rebellious." Cheech remarked that he could now buy weed "from a store in a strip mall," whereas before he could only buy it from "behind a store in a strip mall."

BOB MARLEY

The Jamaican reggae legend was a Rastafarian who revered ganja as a so-called sacramental herb. Though Marley is widely viewed as a pot smoker, he used the drug not recreationally but for religious and meditative purposes. In an interview with biographer Stephen Davis, Marley said, "Rastaman sit down and smoke some herb, with good meditation, and a policeman come see him, stick him up, search him, beat him, and put him in prison. Now, what is this guy doing these things for? Herb grows like yams and cabbage. Just grow. Policemen do these things for evil."

CHELSEA HANDLER

This American comedian often talks publicly about her marijuana use. In fact, in September 2018 she launched a seven-city tour to discuss marijuana, politics, and comedy. She delved deeper into cannabis use recently for sleep issues, but mostly she enjoys the drug for its calming effect and says she likes giggling with her girlfriends after consuming edibles. The outspoken comedian mused publicly in February 2018 on

Instagram that she had thoughts of growing her own line of weed, to be sold in micro-doses and marketed to women. In September 2018 she told a reporter for the *Leaf*, a Canadian cannabis news outlet, "I think it's great, I think I've seen it change people in my life. I want people to know about it. . . . And it's helped me so much [to] cope, and actually do much more good work, and have the patience not to blow my gasket every morning when I wake up and read the news."

JUSTIN TIMBERLAKE

The American singer, songwriter, actor, dancer, record producer, athlete, and heartthrob was quoted in *Playboy* magazine in 2011 discussing how pot allows him to stop thinking and just be. "Sometimes I have a brain that just needs to be turned off," he said, likely referring to his ADHD and OCD diagnoses. "Some people are just better high."

SUSAN SARANDON

The 72-year-old Academy Award and Screen Actors Guild Award winning actress and liberal activist has a penchant for weed and isn't afraid to discuss it. This celebrated film, TV, and Broadway star has smoked pot recreationally since her college days and has admitted to being high at most major industry award shows that she attends. In a 2014 interview with reporter Marlow Stern of the *Daily Beast*, Sarandon said, "People don't get mean on weed, don't beat up their wives on weed, and don't drive crazy on weed. They just get hungry." Two years later she explained to host Andy Cohen on Bravo's *Watch What Happens Live* her attitude about limits with marijuana: "When you can't find the joint that you lit, it's probably time to stop."

TV Shows and Movies Cannabisseurs Love

> "Have you ever looked at the back of a dollar bill . . . ooon weeeed?"
> —Jon Stewart in *Half-Baked*

As Jon Stewart's character, Enhancement Smoker, points out in the 1998 stoner film *Half-Baked*, everything is better on weed. If you're looking for some quality home or theatrical entertainment, the following TV shows and movies definitely get better with a nice high. Though this is not comprehensive, you will find plenty of recommendations that should be at the top of your list. (Plus the best stoner quotes from each.)

CLASSIC STONER MOVIES

If the main character is a stoner, then clearly you're in the right place. Here is your must-see short list.

Up in Smoke (1978)

Man: "You wanna get high, man?"

Pedro: "Does Howdy Doody got wooden balls, man?"

Harold and Kumar Go to White Castle (2004)

Harold: "Dude, we're so high right now."
Kumar: "We're not low!"

Half-Baked (1998)

Thurgood Jenkins: "I don't do drugs though. Just weed."

Dazed and Confused (1993)

Wooderson: "Say, man, you got a joint?"
Mitch: "No, not on me, man."
Wooderson: "It'd be a lot cooler if you did."

Friday (1995)

Smokey: "Weed is from the earth. God put this here for me and you. Take advantage, man, take advantage."

The Big Lebowski (1998)

The Dude: "Walter, I love you, but sooner or later, you're going to have to face the fact you're a goddamn moron."

SETH ROGEN, JAMES FRANCO, AND JONAH HILL MOVIES

This category features a great combination of a modern subset of stoner movies, hilarious comedies, and instant classics. Although these actors have had a hand in a number of incredible films, Franco's *127 Hours* is worth skipping, unless you're looking for reasons to be super paranoid. The top of the list includes:

Pineapple Express (2008)

Saul: "It's almost a shame to smoke it. It's like killing a unicorn . . . with, like, a bomb."

This Is the End (2013)

Jonah Hill: "Weed is tight . . . weed is tight."

22 Jump Street (2014)

Schmidt: "Slam . . . poetry. Yelling! Angry! Waving my hands a LOT! Specific point of view on THINGS! Cynthia! Cyn-thi-a! Jesus died for our sin-thi-as! Jesus cried, runaway bride. Julia Roberts! Julia Rob . . . hurts! Cynthia! Ooh, Cynthia. You're dead. You are dead. Bop boop beep bop bop boop bop. You're dead. That's for Cynthia . . . who's dead."

The Wolf of Wall Street (2013)

Jordan Belford: "The first thing we needed was brokers. Guys with sales experience. So I recruited some of my hometown boys: Sea Otter, who sold meat and weed; Chester, who sold tires and weed; and Robbie, who sold anything he could get his hands on . . . mostly weed."

Knocked Up (2007)

Ben Stone: "You know, the best thing for a hangover is weed. Do you smoke weed?"

Superbad (2007)

Officer: "How old are you, McLovin?"
Fogell: "Old enough."
Officer: "Old enough for what?"
Fogell: "To party."

CLASSIC COMEDIES

Good comedies become laugh-out-loud comedies with the enhancement of an herbal refreshment. The list is endless, but here are a few favorites that won't disappoint.

Ted (2012)

Narrator: "Now if there's one thing you can be sure of, it's that nothing is more powerful than a young boy's wish. Except an Apache helicopter. An Apache helicopter has machine guns AND missiles. It is an unbelievably impressive complement of weaponry, an absolute death machine."

Anchorman: The Legend of Ron Burgundy (2004)

Brian Fantana: "They've done studies, you know. Sixty percent of the time, it works every time."

Fast Times at Ridgemont High (1982)

Desmond: "That kid's been stoned since the third grade."

Office Space (1999)

Peter Gibbons: "The thing is, Bob, it's not that I'm lazy, it's that I just don't care."

Airplane! (1980)

Elaine: "Ladies and gentlemen, this is your stewardess speaking. We regret any inconvenience the sudden cabin movement might have caused; this is due to periodic air pockets we encountered. There's no reason to become alarmed, and we hope you enjoy the rest of your flight. By the way, is there anyone on board who knows how to fly a plane?"

National Lampoon's Van Wilder (2002)

Dad: "Where can I find Van Wilder?"
Wasted Guy: "In the Guinness Book of World Fucking Records, man. Under Raddest Fucking Dude Alive!"

TRIPPY MOVIES

Each entry on this list might include a classic trippy scene, or the entire movie might feel like one intensely long voyage. Regardless, the best part about watching these movies stoned is that you won't remember much of the plot. So seeing them a second time is just as good. (For the ultimate trippy movie/music experience, see page 136.)

Fight Club (1999)

Tyler Durden: "Gentlemen, welcome to Fight Club. The first rule of Fight Club is you do not talk about fight club. The second rule of fight club is you DO NOT talk about Fight Club!"

Memento (2000)

Leonard: "I take it I've told you about my condition."
Teddy: "Only every time I see ya."

Fear and Loathing in Las Vegas (1998)

Raoul Duke: "We had two bags of grass, seventy-five pellets of mescaline, five sheets of high-powered blotter acid, a salt shaker half full of cocaine, and a whole galaxy of multicolored uppers, downers, screamers, laughers . . . Also, a quart of tequila, a quart of rum, a case of beer, a pint of raw ether, and two dozen amyls. Not that we needed all that for the trip, but once you get locked into a serious drug collection, the tendency is to push it as far as you can."

Inception (2010)

Cobb: "Dreams feel real while we're in them. It's only when we wake up that we realize something was actually strange."

Magnolia (1999)

Jimmy Gator: "The book says, 'We might be through with the past, but the past ain't through with us.'"

HOW TO WATCH *THE WIZARD OF OZ* WHILE LISTENING TO PINK FLOYD'S *DARK SIDE OF THE MOON*

1. Set *The Wizard of Oz* to play, preferably with subtitles turned on. Lower or mute the volume.

2. Prepare *The Dark Side of the Moon* to play on repeat on your turntable or preferred music player.

3. Start *The Wizard of Oz*. When the MGM lion roars for the third time during the opening title credits, start *The Dark Side of the Moon*.

4. To confirm that the film and album are in sync, the music should transition from "Speak to Me" to "Breathe" when the "Produced by Mervyn Leroy" credit appears on the screen.

5. Kick back and enjoy the curious synchronicity.

ACTION MOVIES

When we watch these movies high, the action can feel quicker and more intense. With this genre, your best bet is to go see the newest releases in 3-D at the theater. But if the couch is where you're at, here are a few to try after a puff or two.

Kill Bill: Vol. 1 (2003)

Budd: "That woman deserves her revenge and we deserve to die."

The Matrix (1999)

Morpheus: "This is your last chance. After this, there is no turning back. You take the blue pill, the story ends, you wake up in your bed and believe whatever you want to believe. You take the red pill, you stay in Wonderland, and I show you how deep the rabbit hole goes."

Kung Fu Hustle (2004)

The Beast: "Don't get me wrong! I only want to kill you, or be killed by you."

300 (2006)

Messenger: "This is madness!"
King Leonidas: "Madness? THIS. IS. SPARTA!!!"

NETFLIX AND CHILLLLLL

This popular streaming service has a ton of programming that can be enjoyed stoned, from mind-blowing thrillers to hilarious comedies. Here are some of the best selections.

Black Mirror (2011–)

This futuristic science-fiction series of stand-alone episodes examines the unintended consequences of technology on humanity.

American Vandal season one (2017)

Imagine if *Making a Murderer* were a documentary about a high-school kid who spray-paints penises on every car in the faculty parking lot. Grab your one-hitter and binge-watch this one.

Sacrifice (2018)

In this 49-minute special, master illusionist Derren Brown creates an intense situation for one American man who possesses strong opinions about illegal immigrants. Don't look up more information about this; just get high and watch it.

Tickled (2016)

This mystery documentary will keep you guessing—and wondering why anyone would tell you to watch it stoned. Sorry, but not sorry.

THE CULTURE OF CANNABIS

DOCUMENTARIES

But I don't watch these when I'm sober, why would I watch them high? Stimulate your mind, my friend, and stop being so negative. Couple the documentaries below with a good smoke, and you will unlock the incredibly complex mysteries of the universe. Or at least you'll think you have.

Samsara (2001)

This film was made in twenty-five countries over five years. There is no narration whatsoever, only extremely trippy visuals set to unique background music.

Cosmos: A Spacetime Odyssey (2014)

Executive producer Seth MacFarlane developed this thirteen-episode documentary hosted by author and astrophysicist Neil deGrasse Tyson. The show will have a dramatic effect on your perspective of the universe and your place in it.

Cave of Forgotten Dreams (2010)

This film takes you back in time about 30,000 years as director Werner Herzog navigates the inside of a cave that contains the oldest recorded paintings by humans.

FUNNY CLASSIC TELEVISION

Laughing is one of the great side effects of marijuana use and provides a great ab workout, too. Old episodes of *The Muppet Show*, *Friends*, *Teen Titans Go!*, and *The Simpsons* can provide just the spark you need to get your body ready for the summer. (The munchies are another side effect, however, so maybe don't break out that swimwear just yet.)

14 Albums Every Cannabisseur Should Know

There is little science about why listening to music stoned can be so satisfying, but the cannabisseur knows there is no comparison for the emotional connection that occurs when music combines with the perfect high. Many musicians have used cannabis, dating all the way back to the jazz scene of the early 1900s. For fans, listening to music while high is a decades-old pastime. Hip-hop, concert jams, reggae, classic rock—there are no rules except to select tunes that best fit the mood you're in or, perhaps, the mood you want to be in.

The cannabisseur remembers to turn the television off once in a while and turn up the tunes. Set the right playlist, hike up the volume, sit back, and enjoy. Here are some of my favorite artists and albums from across the musical spectrum to listen to with a joint in hand. If you read this list and blurt out how absurd it is that D'Angelo wasn't included, it is recommended that you go get high and relax.

- *Bizarre Ride II the Pharcyde* by the Pharcyde (1992)
- *The Dark Side of the Moon* by Pink Floyd (1973)

- *Doggystyle* by Snoop Dogg (1993)
- *Enter the Wu-Tang (36 Chambers)* by Wu-Tang Clan (1993)
- *Exodus* by Bob Marley and the Wailers (1977)
- *40 Oz. to Freedom* by Sublime (1992)
- *Led Zeppelin IV* by Led Zeppelin (1971)
- *Live/Dead* by Grateful Dead (1969)
- *More Life* by Drake (2017)
- *Paranoid* by Black Sabbath (1970)
- *Remain in Light* by Talking Heads (1980)
- *Rift* by Phish (1993)
- *2001* by Dr. Dre (1999)
- *Voodoo* by D'Angelo (2000)*

*There, are you happy?

Further Reading

Pot Culture: The A–Z Guide to Stoner Language and Life
by Shirley Halperin and Steve Bloom

The Cannabis Grow Bible: The Definitive Guide to Growing Marijuana for Recreational and Medicinal Use
by Greg Green

Cannabis Pharmacy: The Practical Guide to Medical Marijuana
by Michael Backes

The Cannabis Encyclopedia: The Definitive Guide to Cultivation & Consumption of Medical Marijuana
by Jorge Cervantes

Leafly
leafly.com

High Times
hightimes.com

PotGuide
potguide.com

The Cannabist
thecannabist.co

Proper
aproperhigh.com

Acknowledgments

My sincere thanks to Brett Cohen for providing me with the opportunity to write this book.

Thank you Jhanteigh Kupihea, Jane Morley, and the entire Quirk Books staff for turning some great ideas into a really fun book.

To my wife, whose love and support I could never live without. To my children, who inspire me and give me hope for our future. To my parents, who taught me more than they will ever know.

To my friends, thanks for making the good times so damn great.